THE LOSERS

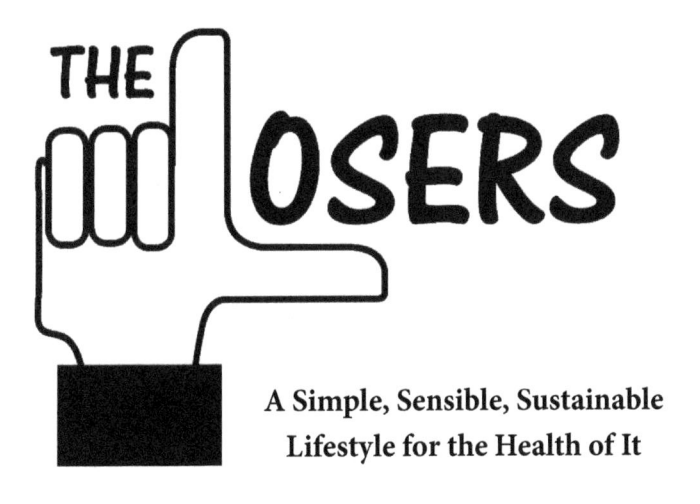

A Simple, Sensible, Sustainable Lifestyle for the Health of It

by Ruby Dillon

Copyright © 2018 by Ruby Dillon

All rights reserved.

No part of this book may be reproduced or transmitted in any form or by any means without written permission from the author.

ISBN 978-1-62806-203-8

Library of Congress Control Number 2018967174

Published by Salt Water Media
29 Broad Street, Suite 104
Berlin, MD 21811
www.saltwatermedia.com

The contents of this book, such as text, graphics, images, information obtained from public domain sources, are for informational purposes only. The content is not intended to be a substitute for professional medical or nutritional advice, diagnosis, or treatment. Always seek the advice of your physician or other qualified health provider with any questions you may have regarding a medical condition or embarking on any weight loss or exercise program that may be mentioned in this book. Use of the information in this book, and the Loser program, is solely at your own risk. Never disregard professional medical advice or delay in seeking it because of something you have read in this book.

I'm going to make you so proud.

-note to self

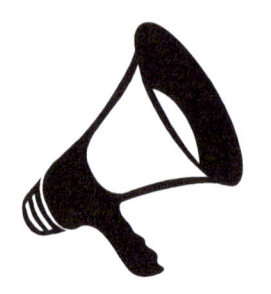

They say 'Diet,'
We say 'LIFESTYLE!'
They say 'Cheat,'
We say 'CHOICES!'
LIFESTYLE, CHOICES!
LIFESTYLE, CHOICES!
Gooooo! LOSERS!

We start each meeting with this cheer because we're glad you're here!

Find us on Facebook!
Just search: Losers Around the World.
Please join us and share your recipes, questions, and inspirations!

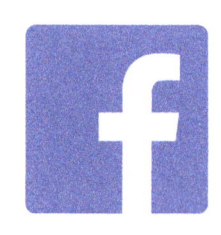

DEDICATION

To my husband, Bob Dillon,
my biggest cheerleader, great shopper, and chef!

And to my family and Loser friends:
You have helped me tremendously
to literally lift a weight off my shoulders.

CONTENTS

Preface 11

Introduction 14

Chapter One: LOSING FOR LOSERS 15

Chapter Two: SUCCESSFUL LOSERS 18

Chapter Three: TRACKING FOR LOSERS 23

Chapter Four: PASSING PLATEAUS FOR LOSERS 27

Chapter Five: EXERCISE FOR LOSERS 30

Afterword 34

Epilogue 37

Addendum 38

Appendix A: Fruit and Losers 39

Appendix B: Lean Protein for Losers 41

Appendix C: Ruby's Pantry 42

Appendix D: Recipes for Losers 45

Appendix E: Tracking Chart for Losers 51

PREFACE

In 2009, I became depressed and disgusted with the way I felt and the way I looked. I didn't have the energy and stamina to be as active as I liked. I was worried about my health. Heart disease and diabetes run in my family and, frankly, I was afraid for my future quality of life. At 52, I shouldn't have had thoughts about my mortality! With the encouragement of my daughter, Susan, we joined a national weight loss program. Two years, four months, and 18 days later I reached my goal weight with 62 pounds lost.

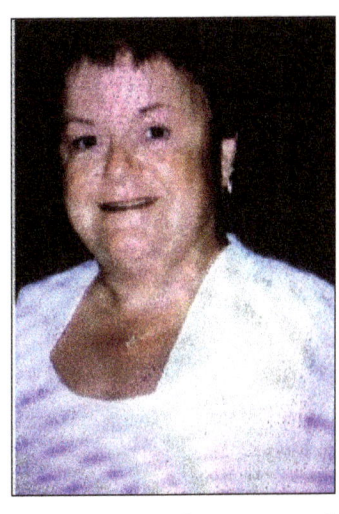

I was so pleased with my accomplishment I wanted to help others who wanted to lose weight, so I joined a national team. I worked for this company for nearly 3 years. During that time, I developed a personal perspective on weight loss and noticed that sticking to a plan worked for some clients and seemed to make no difference for others. Maybe it was the client's interpretation, or misinterpretation, of the plan?

I know, for me, I was modifying the plan in order to stop losing weight and maintain what I had lost. Maybe that was the difference, doing something beyond just following a plan. By then it was time to go a different way in order to help others who found that a national plan wasn't making the difference in their lives that they wanted.

Although I had no nutritional background, nor a degree

in nutrition, I knew I did have a lot of common sense. I truly learned from experience what was necessary - adapting to a lifestyle of healthier eating and better choices to lose and maintain weight loss.

I knew that no one became overweight by eating too much lean protein or too many non-starchy vegetables. What makes us fat are too many carbohydrates and too many fats. So, what was the magic number that would help us lose weight and develop a lifestyle that could last forever?

With the help of nutritional articles, the internet and other people's experiences, I developed the LOSER program. I introduced the program in 2014 with an ad in the local newspaper and announced it to my friends. I am thrilled that it was so well received and that our members have seen positive results that meet their personal lifestyle.

I have included charts throughout the book to show how this is a simple tracking program with flexibility! I cannot stress enough that there is nothing you cannot eat; you just have to plan for it.

I also knew that no one can eat unlimited amounts of fruit (i.e. – bananas, pineapple, and watermelon, etc.) without it interfering with losing weight. That is because fruits are filled with carbohydrates in the form of sugars! Losers understand that they need to track fruit. It is not a "freebie" food.

The Loser program is not a quick weight loss diet. It is meant for you to lose slow and steady as your mindset and lifestyle changes, which is truly needed to be successful. The Loser program does not cut out anything from your diet. It is a GREAT guideline to make choices regarding the food you want to eat, after all, YOU know your body and mind.

Once you understand "forever," you accept there is no race to a goal, because there really never is a goal. You must be JOURNEY HAPPY, not destination happy.

It's also important to remember, that NO ONE should ever be hungry or bored!

Ruby Dillon, Loser

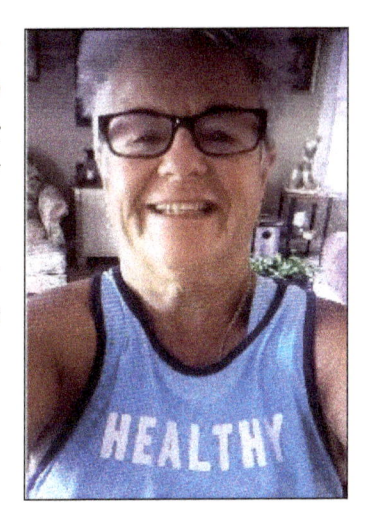

INTRODUCTION

This is an age-friendly health program. Losers are motivated at different stages in their lives. Losers range in age from their 20's to their 80's, there are no age limits. Losers come in all shapes and sizes, but there are no weight limits. Losers may have some limitations or no limitations, it doesn't matter. Losers lose weight at different rates, but whether rapidly or steadily, **all Losers lose**!

Losers have fun. Losers encourage others. Loser meetings are judgement-free zones. Losers are sincerely pleased by the accomplishment of others. Everyone can be a Loser.

> *"We are on a forever journey and we're all human. So, when we slip and gain some there is never any judgment - everyone else has also been there and done that. We simply encourage each other and Loser support is the best! We're all on this journey together."*
>
> *- Mary Lou*

CHAPTER ONE: LOSING FOR LOSERS

> "You taught us a lot about Fats and Carbs, also how you must read nutrition labels. We also felt relaxed to express our thoughts and how we felt about things to do with The LOSERS Group."
>
> - Clarence

The Loser way to managing your food intake is tracking Net Carbohydrates (total carbohydrates minus the amount of fiber) and total Fat grams. I developed this form of tracking because the Loser program needed something simpler than calorie counting, games, and fad diets. On a daily basis I track approximately 130grams (g) of Net Carbohydrates (NC) and 30g of Fat. It is working wonderfully and it's so much simpler. Not only have I kept off the 62 pounds I lost seven years ago, but I've found it easier to maintain a lower weight and eat healthy and tasteful foods.

Tracking NCs encourages fiber filled eating. You must track fruit under NC, so you don't "over fruit." Appendix B is a chart listing some common fruits and their NCs.

> "I tried to diet and only found it to be a rollercoaster of up and down weight. Each time it was up, it was higher than the last time. Ruby supplied the information I needed to select foods that made sense while not depriving myself as a 'diet' often did. With Ruby's ongoing support and education, she has made it easy for me to eat right while slowly and steadily losing weight! My health is better, my doctor no longer considers me a diabetic, I am off all medications, and I feel so much better. The Loser program has changed my whole way of thinking and eating. This is a lifestyle I can live with!"
>
> - Joan

Read nutrition labels! And don't forget to look at the serving size on the label – if you're using the full container, multiply the NC and the total Fat by the number of servings of that container.

Losers consider calories, but Losers don't track calories. Why? You can reach your calorie limit quickly by eating cake or chips. But tracking NCs and Fats encourages you to select healthier, satisfying foods while keeping the simplicity of the program. Adding to the simplicity is that there are only three lifestyle groups for Losers: 130/30, 140/40, and 150/50 (Daily total for Net Carbs/Daily total for Fat).

Use nutrition labels to determine how many grams of fat are present in your favorite foods. Or, use an online nutrition database – such as the U.S. Department of Agriculture's National Nutrient Database – to figure out how many grams of fat you're eating daily.

A nutrition label gives you all the information you need to easily track fat and carbohydrates.

> *"This is by far the simplest way to get the best results... and all you have to do is read... and do a few calculations... carbs – fiber = Net Carbs... total your Fats and NCs daily... easy peasy!"*
>
> *- Laura*

> *"I was a stress eater. As a family caregiver under frequent stress, I would eat. Now I use a time-out and think about whether I am hungry or if it is just stress. The Loser program is helping me make better food choices all the time!"*
>
> *- Pat*

Read the Label!

TOTAL CARBS
minus
DIETARY FIBER
equals
NET CARBS
per serving

A health bar can be a drive-through alternative for a healthy snack!

Read the label and make a choice! For example, according to this label, one cup is only 4 grams of Fat and 31 NCs!

Nutrition Facts

Serving Size 1 Cup
Servings Per Container 5

Amount Per Serving

Calories 310

% Daily Value

Total Fat 4g	**5%**
Saturated Fat 0g	0%
Trans Fat 0g	0%
Cholesterol 0mg	**0%**
Sodium 200mg	**10%**
Total Carbohydrate 36g	**15%**
Dietary Fiber 5g	17%
Total Sugars 13g	13%
Protein 10g	
Vitamin D 4mcg	
Calcium 227mg	
Iron 8mg	
Potassium 159mg	

CHAPTER TWO: SUCCESSFUL LOSERS

✔ **ALL YOU CARE to EAT**

✘ **ALL YOU CAN to EAT**

First - The "Ville"

Everyone has a "happy place in life." Some of us have a few. For me, I find comfort in certain stores and I return often, and there are some vacation destinations that are happy places that I visit often. I came to discover that another happy place for me was when I followed a plan for eating, exercising, and losing weight. I started calling this place where I was so happy, "The Ville." No particular reason, it just seems like a quaint and happy name and especially a nice place to live. And so, it was born. A place to come home to if I visited "Eating Land" longer than I wanted to.

Now, after a vacation or a holiday where I may have over indulged it always feels good to go BACK TO THE VILLE.

Losers often give an encouraging word with a smile to any of the Losers we pass and add the greeting, "Stay in the Ville!"

Directions to the Ville

The Loser program is a progressive weight loss program. Many who adopt the program are overweight because they overeat and they are used to eating more. Their stomach has expanded to accommodate the volume of food they are used to eating. Taking into account that reducing the size of your stomach contributes to success, Losers can choose at what stage they want to begin their lifestyle journey. Those who are more than 50 pounds overweight have a larger stomach size and if they cut back too soon they usually "crash" and have to deal with feelings of deprivation or physical hunger. Starting with a greater NetCarb/Fat ratio helps them steadily lose weight and gives their stomach time to begin to shrink. Once they have reached a stage where they are less than 50 pounds above their target weight they adjust their NetCarb/Fat ratio to the next lower level.

For example, if a Loser begins less than 25 pounds over where they would like to be, they would consume no more than 130 grams of NCs and 30 grams of Fat per day because their stomach is probably closer to a reasonable size. To lose 25-50 pounds they would start by limiting their NC and Fat ratio to 140/40, because their stomach needs to shrink. If a person is more than 50 pounds from their target weight, because they are used to a larger volume of food per day, they should start with a ratio of no more than 150 NCs and 50 grams Fat per day. These can be adjusted as you drop weight.

Pounds to Lose	Daily Maximum Net-Carb Grams	Daily Maximum Fat Grams
<25	130	30
25 - 50	140	40
>50 or more	150	50

Losers track the Fat and NCs daily. Sometimes a Loser will leave the Ville for various reasons for a day or two or a weekend. Getting back to the Ville is easy – new day, new track.

The Loser lifestyle is planning ahead. One big step is reading labels or searching for the nutritional values for Fat and NCs BEFORE you order the "salad" – which, in some restaurants, based on its contents can use up your total fat and/or Net-Carbs for the day! Say What!?! "But it's a salad!").

> "A diet has an expiration date, a lifestyle doesn't."
> - Kathe Hoban, nutritionist

If you know you're going to an event that might send you over the limit for the day, then plan accordingly. Make up the difference by modifying your choices a few days before or a few days after the event. It's easier to have fun knowing that you planned for the event and that you know how to "get back to the Ville." Remember, the Loser program is a lifestyle, not a diet. So, plan ahead and enjoy that tailgate party, you are always welcome back to the Ville!

> "When I started as a Loser, I didn't want to beat myself up if I went over my daily 150/50 limit. So, I tracked daily to begin teaching myself how to plan and/or make up for a bad day at some other point DURING THE WEEK. I focused on a weekly "daily average" and if the average was not over 150/50 a day – I was making progress. It wasn't long before I was able to more accurately get to "know" and "live" at 150/50 or less a day.
>
> - James

What about alcohol? We have no real rules about it, but this is what I've learned and know. When we drink alcoholic beverages we often become weaker about making good food choices. When I do choose to drink, I don't drink the high sugar drinks like margaritas or orange crushes, or sugary shots like a fireball. Each day that I expect to drink alcohol I also eat spot on, drink lots of water, and get more exercise than usual. It's all about "finding your balance."

> The longer you are a Loser, you develop most often without realizing it, a positive mindset and perspective about food. Not as a negative associated with weight, but as a positive associated with lifestyle. Losers choose the lifestyle they prefer and make the choices necessary to achieve it. YOU ARE IN CONTROL.

Losers also find substitutes for an alcoholic drink or drink a non-alcoholic beverage between alcoholic ones. It is important to discover a new zero calorie drink that you enjoy. I love a large colorful glass with iced tea or Vitamin Zero water, the lemon flavor. Other favorites are Club Soda with a few fresh limes. Find yours!

Keep on Tracking!

Well meaning friends and family, and those who don't understand the Loser program, can be a challenge. Keep in mind that they may make suggestions but you make the choices. You decide what you want to put into your mouth even when you can't choose what goes onto your plate. This is your health and you should tactfully give it a priority.

I also have said to members, when they get all freaky about company coming, that your guests need to "respect your kitchen."

The best thing I ever did was explain to my girlfriends who, for 9 years, had been visiting me from New York and bringing bagels and pastries as a "treat." I asked them to please stop! At first, they couldn't believe I wanted to end this tradition. When they visited for the tenth year, I was determined to let them see *and* taste how great I eat and that I was losing weight! That convinced them. And they follow the Loser program from New York and each one has done amazing!

> "NO" is a complete sentence.

CHAPTER THREE: TRACKING FOR LOSERS

Many Losers have grown up with the familiar four basic food groups (fruit/vegetables, milk, meat, and cereal/bread) established in 1956. Since 1990 the number of food groups have ranged from the basic four up to 11! The latest Department of Health and Human Services and Department of Agriculture *2015 – 2020 Dietary Guidelines for Americans*, 8th Edition, identifies 6 food groups. It's enough to confuse you. Luckily, Losers don't track food groups. Losers track Net Carbohydrates and Fat in the food they choose to eat. That's all. Simple.

> Everything in life is a reflection of a choice you have made. If you don't like your life, make different choices.
> - Anonymous

Losers are encouraged to make nutritional choices, within the food groups they select, to meet their self-determined number of NCs and Fat grams that they choose to eat each day.

You MUST track all of the foods that are trackable. Here lies the simplicity because you won't be tracking any lean protein (lean protein is 93% fat free or greater) or clean (no added fat) non-starchy vegetables (but we do track the starchy vegetables like corn, peas, potatoes, legumes, etc.). Nor do you need to track calorie free drinks.

Keeping a daily record of what you consume each day is important so that you begin to understand what you are actually eating and how much. Everything matters.

> "We are NOT on a diet! We are living a healthy and easy to manage lifestyle. Reducing carbs and fats, Losers have lost weight and manage to keep it off. This is a program that is easy to follow with proven results!"
>
> — Linda

Regarding eggs, if you eat 1-3 as your main source of protein at a meal, cooked clean, we do NOT track them. However, if you choose to snack on them (such as a hard-boiled egg, you need to track 5 Fats).

Do Losers track body weight and measurements? These statistics help you to determine your progress, but that would be your choice. At Losers meetings, members can volunteer to be weighed (it's kept private) but weighing in is not a requirement. It's your choice!

Here are some tips on how to keep a daily tracker chart:

Tracking Tips

- I let the LEAN protein (93% or greater lean), or no more than 2.5 fat grams per ounce and smart vegetables (no added Fat) take care of themselves. *No need to track lean protein.*
- A net carb is total carb minus fiber.
- Track fruit under the net carbs column.
- Anything without a label, simply google "nutrition of <food>" and you can get the nutritional information.
- No guessing.
- Read all nutrition labels and track it.

- Use a small notebook with 3 columns to record your intake: Food, Net Carb, and Fat. A sample page is shown in Appendix A.
- You can use on-line electronic tracking programs like "My Fitness Pal," and most programs and apps have free versions.
- Drink plenty of water.
- Exercise. If you are not doing anything, do something.
- Don't skip breakfast.

Why is it important to track? Because to make wise lifestyle decisions you have to have the best information and facts. Tracking increases your knowledge and helps you pay attention to what's important. Example: Do you know that those "healthy almonds" you often reach for have 18 Fats in 1 ounce? Can you have them? Sure, if you think they're worth it! Just plan ahead to include them in your daily fat target. Choices!

When you have guests with kids, sometimes it is hard to avoid a drive-through snack or meal. Unfortunately, most Fast Foods are fat foods. It is easy to forget that some menu items can blow your entire day. It is hard to plan for a spontaneous drive-through visit. Even a single chicken burger can be 25 grams of fat and 40 grams of net carbs. A sausage-egg-cheese biscuit can be 49 grams of fat and 36 grams of net carbs. And an extra crispy chicken breast is 33 grams of fat and 16 grams of net carbohydrates. If you think a drive-through meal is

> *What I realized as a Loser is I was mindlessly digging my grave with a fork.*
> — Mike

in your future, check this link to find out what choices you can make that you'll feel comfortable with. Losers learn to have a healthy/smart snack with them at all times so they are prepared when a hungry moment may hit them.

https://fastfoodnutrition.org/fast-food-restaurants

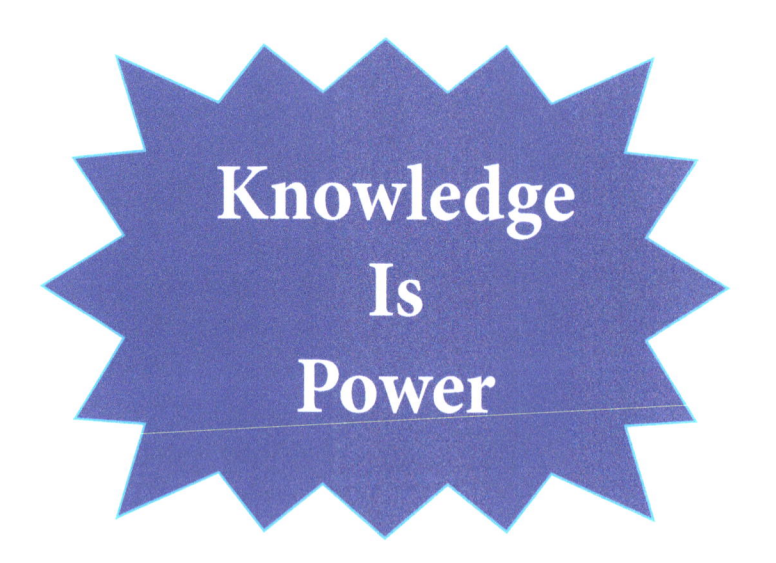

Knowledge Is Power

CHAPTER FOUR: PASSING PLATEAUS FOR LOSERS

Sometimes during a weight loss program there comes a time when losing weight slows down or stops. This is referred to as a plateau.

Always keep in mind that the scale is NOT the only way to measure success. Other ways to gauge how you are doing include:
1. Clothes becoming looser.
2. Measuring tape – Take your measurements at the start of your journey and periodically during it to see your progress.
3. Photographs – periodically take a selfie or have a trusted friend take photos so you can truly see your progress.

> *"This is the easiest program ever! We eat great, we can be creative, and we actually lose weight. Knowledge is the power!"*
> *- Debbie*

Loser's tips for Busting through a Plateau
- Honesty in your tracking – weighing and measuring. We are bad guessers and great pretenders.
- Timeliness in your tracking. We have terrible memories at the end of the day, track as you go.
- Eat more lean protein (beauty of The Losers, we

don't track lean protein!)
- Don't reward exercise with poor choices of food.
- Change up your daily menu, your body gets bored with the same foods.
- Periodically take a break from the Ville foods.
- It may simply be time to move to a lower level of NetCarb/Fat ratio.

General tips for general health and well-being
- Reduce your carb intake in this order: processed foods and then non-processed food. (Example: Choose to eat a potato before choosing to eat potato chips.)
- 7-8 hours of sleep per night.
- Drink more water.
- Cut back on salt.
- Move more (park far, take stairs at work, etc.)
- Manage your alcohol intake.
- Change up your exercise routine.
- Eat regularly, never be hungry. So, if you're really hungry, have that second chicken breast, pork chop, or lean hamburger. There's no tracking it!

> You may see me struggle, but you'll never see me quit.
> - Louis D'Alto

Why Losers are Successful
We share a lot of similarities, particularly successful Losers.
- We are patient. We understand that a total target weight loss does not happen overnight or in a week or sometimes even months. We will see

weight loss, that's for sure, and understand that we are changing our lifestyle and are not on a diet.

• We make choices. We don't make major and radical changes to our nutrition. We track and adjust. We don't stop eating or reduce the number of meals we eat in a day, that's just nonsense and not healthy.

• We reward ourselves, but not with food. A food treat works for training animals, but Losers treat themselves to an outing, a date night, an addition to their wardrobe, etc.

> If you never quit, then you never have to start over.

• We keep in touch. In today's social media world, a Loser is never alone. There is always someone to support them. Because the Loser lifestyle is easy, a lot of support come from their own families. Losers support one another and attending meetings is proven to help Losers stay in the Ville!

• We recognize that our primary goal is better health and longevity.

• We are realistic. Losers know that occasionally they will leave the Ville, but they know they can always come back. Sometimes life throws you a curve and a Loser can be emotionally stressed just like everyone else. Take care of yourself and you will know when it's time to go back to the Ville. A successful Loser never moves permanently away from the Ville.

CHAPTER 5:
EXERCISE FOR LOSERS

You can lose weight without exercise, but only if you also pay attention to the nutrition you are putting into your body. There is certainly a connection between weight loss and exercise. Many nutritionists, fitness coaches, and other health professionals describe the connection with weight loss as 80% of what you eat and 20 % of how you exercise. I have found that it is absolutely imperative to remember, "You cannot out exercise a bad diet."

> You either have a reason or you have an excuse.

The Loser program focus is on the fat that is created when your body consumes more food than it needs. The excess food gets converted to fat and stored away in your liver and muscles. How does your body get rid of the fat you are carrying around? When your body needs more energy than it needs to function, it starts a chemical process that converts fat into glucose and it also breaks it down into carbon dioxide and water. The carbon dioxide is exhaled and the water is expelled as tears, sweat, or urine.

The only way to increase the amount of energy your body needs to function is to increase your metabolism, which you do by moving your muscles. Just getting out of bed in the morning and going through your morning routine doubles your metabolic rate, going for a walk triples your metabolic rate,

> It's you versus you. Don't ever forget that.

even doing household chores can triple your metabolism. The more you increase your activity beyond its resting rate, your metabolism will increase and fat will be converted. An added benefit is your metabolism can remain elevated for 10 to 72 hours after you stop exercising, depending on the exercise.

Exercise does NOT have to be anything too organized or done for long periods of time. You don't have to become a workout warrior. I encourage anyone who is not currently exercising to start small. Even if that means setting your kitchen timer to five minutes and then walking around your house. Often you will find that you want to go five more.

> No one ever finishes exercising and says, "Boy, that was a waste of time."

Walking is the most underrated, and absolutely free, exercise you can get. Why not walk, or at least stand up, when you talk on the phone?

Many health professionals have adopted the arbitrary goal of walking 10,000 steps each day. The non-scientific origin of that goal seems to be the result of marketing efforts of companies that were selling pedometers. It just "caught on" and became a standard goal.

However, many more health professionals, and Losers, encourage people to walk at least more than they are currently walking and also take into consideration their ability to exercise within any limitations they might have.

> Losing weight is hard; being overweight is hard. Choose your hard.

> *One Loser literally hated to exercise. He added exercise to his lifestyle by simply treating his daily 30 minutes of exercise the same as a doctor's appointment. He wouldn't miss a doctor's appointment, so, now he doesn't miss his exercise appointment. It didn't matter he was 66 when he discovered his appointment motivation, it matters that he started.*

Exercise is good for oxygen and blood flow to the brain. It is good for increasing lung capacity, and it is a definite mood enhancer.

People who are physically active live longer and have a lower risk of heart disease, stroke, type 2 diabetes, depression, and some cancers, according to the Centers for Disease Control and Prevention (CDC) 2008 Physical Activity Guidelines for Americans.

Weight bearing exercise also helps increase bone strength. As we age we are more susceptible to bone loss and osteoporosis. Including strength training in your exercise routine is an important way to both strengthen bones and increase metabolism. This can be done very simply with the addition of some light weights or stretch bands. Believe it or not, another exercise that helps increase bone strength is . . . walking!

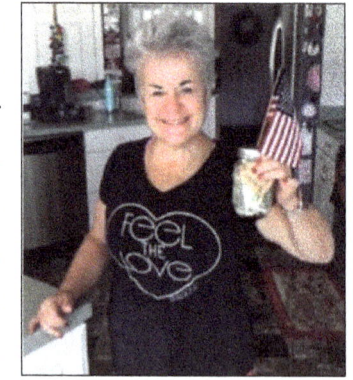

Over 3 years ago I came across an idea how to motivate myself to exercise. It stated that if you keep some sort of jar visible and reward yourself each time you exercise you might just do it more often. My decision was to put $1.00 in a jar each time I walked/ran for at least 3 miles, attended a work out class, or did an at-home workout video for at least 30 minutes. Each time the jar had $100 I would use it to buy some exercise clothes or shoes. I have collected over $250 every year for 3 years now and I am still at it for the 4th year! The best part about this is to remember "your jar, your rules!" Put a penny in or put a marble in; make your requirements a simple 10-minute walk or exercise to a 15-minute video. The whole idea is to move more, and I promise you'll be very proud as that jar fills up.

There are great workout DVDs available, if you are unable to get to a gym, so you can work out right at home. Your cable company might also have exercise programs as part of their basic service package. I am also fond of a website, "Jessicasmithtv.com" because it is a free online site and there are hundreds of workouts that are as short as 8 minutes! Some low impact, some no equipment, some just walking, yoga, stretching and more! YouTube is also a great source for a wide variety of exercise videos. Joining a gym is a great way to meet new friends and be a part of a group class. When you are having fun, you are more apt to keep at it. If you haven't found an exercise you love, then keep looking!

> If you feel like quitting, then think about why you started.

Exercise is a great way to relieve stress and it can often take the place of stress eating! NEVER underestimate exercise!!

AFTERWORD

I was raised by a family of eaters. My immediate family loved to eat, my extended family loved to eat, and being part of an Italian clan meant all holidays and celebrations were focused around food. Looking back, the saddest part of the scenario is that no one tried to make it any better for me so that I wasn't a fat kid. All food in the house was high test. Cookies were an acceptable breakfast, salami sandwiches were an acceptable lunch, and meals were always high in fat and carbs. Second and third helpings were not frowned upon.

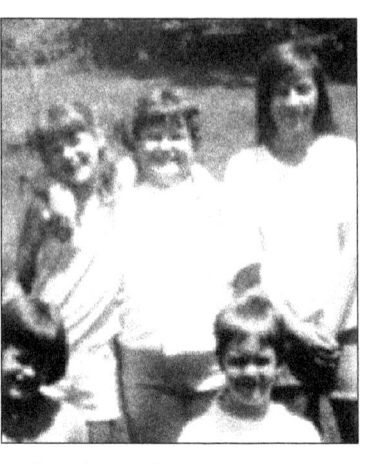

Where's Ruby? In case you need a hint, I'm the one in the center of the photo.

I wasn't made fun of a lot, but often enough. A "moooo" as I walked down the hall at school, or a comment "you have such a cute face, too bad you're so fat," eroded my self-esteem. Probably what stands out the most are three things: (1) the humiliation of having to shop in the "Chubette" department of the store (literally there was a huge sign that hung from the ceiling that said just that). (2) my mother taking me to Take Off Pounds Sensibly (TOPS) meetings and having to stand up and sing "The Pig Song", which included "oinking" whenever you gained weight. (3) In 4th grade the teacher asking the rest of the class how many hotdogs they thought I could eat.

In high school I wore the largest size possible for the gym

romper, which meant the length had to be tailored. Snarky comments were made that additional money had to be spent on me. In the mid 70's it was a lonely dating world for the fat girl. Fat girls didn't get invited to prom, and no kids went alone, totally taboo, so I stayed home. I did get involved in other activities with school clubs and was even awarded most school spirit of the Class of 74'.

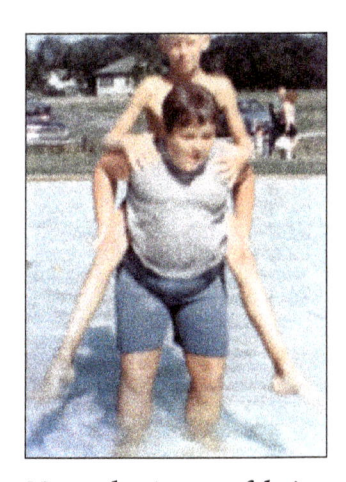

Now, the irony of being the carrier of the "Piggyback" rider is not lost on me. Then it was all about being included.

I worked four summers at a YMCA day camp where I made a best friend. Her mom was a home economics teacher and they had a huge garden on their property. I vividly remember feeling sad for her when she had a lunch that typically included a turkey sandwich on whole wheat bread, carrot sticks, fresh green beans, and an apple. There I sat with my bologna sandwich, potato chips, and a ring ding thinking just how lucky I was. She was always slender and still is today. If I only knew then what I know now.

By now the damage was done. Food was my comfort and my friend. I turned to it when I was happy and especially when I was sad.

So, as you can see I am especially concerned about overweight children. Parents don't realize how hard it will be on them as they grow. Clothes shopping, activities, social development, self-esteem and confidence, and most importantly the foundation of their future health will be a challenge for them to change as an adult. Overweight children have the same health problems as older adults and are seven times more likely to be obese as adults.

In my experience, parents are reluctant to accept their child might be overweight or even obese and they aren't prepared to help them emotionally or nutritionally. When I am approached by a parent I tell them, "your child eats what you bring into the house and what you prepare for them. As you learn about the Loser program you can apply it at home. Chances are your family will never know they are on a weight loss program."

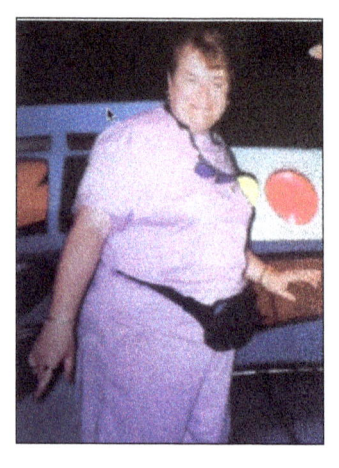

My addiction to food never got better because I just didn't realize all the harm being done to me not only mentally but physically.

That would all change when I turned 52. Better late than never.

> Actually, I just woke up one day and decided
> I didn't want to feel like that anymore,
> or ever again. So I changed.
> Yeah. Just like that.
> - Anonymous

EPILOGUE

Losers is a common-sense approach to losing weight and keeping it off!

FOREVER IN THE VILLE!

"YAY FOR YOU!"

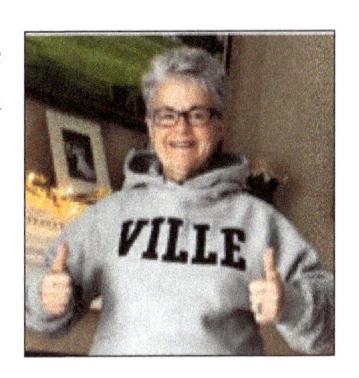

Our meetings begin with our Loser cheer. And I end our meetings with "Broadway Quality Entertainment!" The following is sung to the tune of "My Way!

And now, the day is here, and so I face this weekly weigh in.
My friends, I'll state this clear, my hope is to become slim.
I cooked amazing meals, I walked 3 miles, almost each day.
But more, much more than this, I lost it my way.
Regrets, I have a few, too many beers of this I mention.
I did what I planned to do and saw it through
with great intentions.
I tracked what I knew to track,
a new white page for every new day.
But more, much more than this, I lost it my way.
Yes, there were times, I'm sure you knew.
When I bit off, more than I should chew.
But through it all, when there was doubt,
I got on track and toughed it out.
I faced it all, and I stood tall, and lost it My Way!

ADDENDUM

I grew up beanpole skinny. I was never a dieter. Nutrition was not a concept I understood. I wasn't unhappy, just slowing down because of weight.

On average, I was putting on 3 or 4 pounds a year. After 30 years, we're talking serious weight – almost 100 pounds. I was in my mid-60s and the dial on the scale steadily crept upward. As I expanded into 3X clothing I figured I had two choices, keep adding 3 or 4 pounds each year or do something about it.

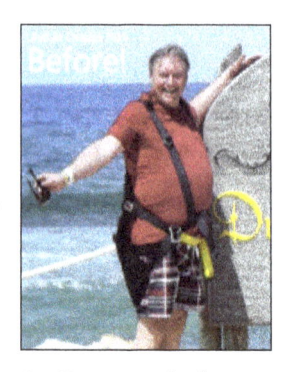

I decided to give losing weight a try but only if I could keep it off. I have friends and family who tried national diets, counselling, and surgery and none of them succeeded in keeping the weight off. And, it had to be simple. I already knew that I was not giving up Happy Hour! A notice in the local newspaper read "Losers. Don't go it alone." I decided to attend, and my wife joined me. The attendees, including other couples, were like us, adults who weren't looking for a diet or rules to reach a weight loss goal. We wanted guidelines. And that's what we got! I lost 13-inches of belly in less than a year and kept it off and moved back to a size L wardrobe. My wife had similar results. And that wasn't all, I came off a lot of medications, stopped needing a C-pap to breathe, and I am in control of my body shape and lifestyle. How did we do it? Easy, we just followed Ruby's Loser program.

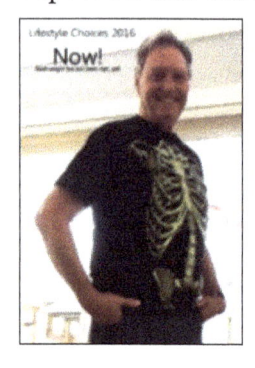

- Tony Kendrick, Loser

APPENDIX A

Fruit with Seeds (1 medium size)	Net Carb
Apple	16
Grape	0.5
Pear	21
Citrus Fruits (1 medium size)	
Grapefruit	18
Lemon	4
Lime	5
Orange	12
Tangerine	10
Stone Fruits (1 medium size)	
Apricot	3
Cherry	1
Nectarine	12
Peach	8
Plum	7
Tropical Fruits (1 medium size)	
Banana	24
Kiwi	9
Coconut (3 oz)	5
Guava	5
Litchis	2
Mangos	32
Papayas	24
Pineapple (3 oz)	9
Melons (1 wedge)	
Cantaloupe	5
Honeydew	10
Watermelon (10 oz)	10

Berries (1 cup)	Net Carb
Blackberries	6
Blueberries	18
Cranberries	8
Raspberries	7
Strawberries	9
Miscellaneous (1 cup)	
Fruit or Fruit Juice Smoothie	31
Fruit and Dairy Smoothie	38
Dried Fruit Mixture	78
Fruit Salad in Light Syrup	36

APPENDIX B

Protein Fats for 4-ounce servings
(lean/Fat trimmed, no marbling, cooked clean)

This chart can be referenced when including these items in your daily tracking log. NOTE: all seafood, as long as it is cooked and prepared clean (no added oils), is considered lean protein. It does NOT need to be tracked.

Protein	Fats*	Protein	Fats*
Lean Deli Roast Beef	4	Filet Mignon	8
Flank Steak	10	Brisket	12
Beef Tenderloin	12.6	Sirloin Steak	12
Skirt Steak	16	Chuck Steak	17
NY Strip Steak	17	T-Bone Steak	18
Flat Iron Steak	19	Ribeye Steak	21
Short Ribs	30	Prime Rib	31
Boneless Pork Chop	4	Ham	4
Tenderloin	6	Sirloin Pork Roast	7
Baby Back Ribs	17	Country Style Ribs	21
Spare Ribs	24	Front Hock	24
Rear Hock	27	Pork Belly	28
Chicken Breast	2.5	Chicken Leg	6.6
Chicken Thigh	12	Turkey Breast	4
Turkey Leg	8	Turkey Thigh	8
Carnival Leg	13	Duck	13
Leg of Veal	4	Lambchop	9

* Good news! If the Fat value is 10 grams or less, you do NOT need to track them, so have a second serving when you're really hungry. If it is greater than 10 grams, you need to track the full value (and not the value minus 10 grams.)

APPENDIX C

A well-stocked kitchen and pantry is the key to success as a Loser.

Included here is what I typically keep in my kitchen at all times. They prove to be not only tasty choices, they have great stats when it comes to lower in Fats and Net Carbs. Lots of veggies and lean protein is at every meal to insure we are never hungry.

I purchase many items in single serving bags. This makes it so easy to carry snacks with me at all times. I find if I am away from home and need something to eat, having it with me prevents me from driving through a fast food restaurant where I might make a poor choice.

Once again, the beauty of the Loser program and the simplicity shines through by you being able to choose just by reading labels!

> The food you eat can be powerful medicine or slow poison.

Solid White Tuna in water pouches
Bulgur Wheat (Red Mill) Quinoa
Polenta (Son of Italy)
Variety of canned red, white, & chic pea beans
Jars of Salsa
Sun dried tomatoes in pouches
No Sodium Chicken and Beef Broth

Lite Soups
Fat Free Cream of Mushroom Soup
Canned tomatoes
Olive Oil
Balsamic Vinegar
Animal Crackers
Large variety of baked chips
Lite Crackers

Sour Dough Pretzel Niblets
Various Mrs. Dash Spices
Sugar Free Jams and Jellies
Cooking Spray
Powdered Peanut Butter (PB2)
Classico Basil & Tomato Pasta Sauce
Low or "90 Calorie" Fiber Bars (2.5F, 12NC)

Low Sodium Roast Beef and Turkey Breast
Eggs and egg whites
Nature's Own Light Honey Wheat Bread
(1F/13NC per 2 slice)
Wrap Up Wraps: (2F/7NC or better)
Extreme Wellness Wraps (1.5F/5NC or better)

Josephs Pitas
Yoplait Greek and regular yogurt
Lite String Cheese
Laughing Cow Light Cheeses
Skim Milk
Land O Lakes Fat Free 1/2 and 1/2
Sugar Free Coffee Mate

Bags of Fresh Express Salad Blends
Lots of seasonal fruits and fresh veggies
Fat Free Jell-O Pudding Cups
Sugar Free Jell-O Cups
Greek Cream Cheese
Small Potatoes

Boneless skinless Chicken Breasts
Salmon Filet
93/7 or Leaner Ground Turkey Breast
95/5 or Leaner Ground Beef

Turkey Tenderloin
Pork Tenderloin
Shrimp
Special K Breakfast Sandwiches
Bags of Chopped Frozen Spinach
Variety of steamable Veggies in Bags
Alexia Potato fries
Boca Burgers
Good Stat Black Bean Burgers
Hershey Kisses
Yasso Frozen Yogurt Bars

> Say "No" once in the store or say "No" often at home until it's all gone.

APPENDIX D

RUBY'S WORLD-FAMOUS TURKEY MEATBALLS
3 Net Carbs and a trace of Fat!
Serving size: 1 meatball
(*Please feel free to add salt, pepper, or any other spice you might like!*)

Ingredients
2 20oz packages of Ground Turkey Breast (93% or leaner)
1 cup Bulgur Wheat (cook first and let cool thoroughly)
6 egg whites
½ cup Grated Parmesan Cheese
6 (or more) cloves of fresh garlic (chopped)
Lots of Fresh Basil

Directions
Combine all ingredients thoroughly. Roll into 40 meatballs. Spray baking dish generously with cooking spray. Put meatballs spaced into dish, you might need two. Spray tops with cooking spray and sprinkle salt lightly on top to add to crispiness and flavor. Bake at 375 degrees for 45 minutes. Turn after 25 minutes so they brown on both sides. Cool and drop in a pot of sauce.

They also freeze great for future meals!

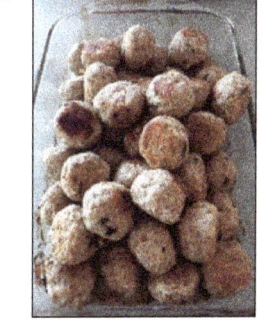

RUBY'S PIZZELLE RECIPE
8 Net Carbs and 1.7 Fat
Serving size: 1 cookie
(yield approximately 13-14 dozen)

Ingredients
7 cups flour
2 cups sugar
2 cups light butter (melt and cool)
8 tsp. baking powder
12 large eggs
3 or 4 tsp. Anis Oil
1 bottle of Anis seeds.

Directions
Beat eggs, light butter, and sugar in large bowl. In a smaller bowl fold baking powder into flour. Gradually add flour mixture into egg mixture. You can use a small mixer. Make sure all lumps are gone. Batter should be thick. Fold in Anis Oil and seeds. Using electric pizzelle iron, spray with a cooking spray. Heat and drop by teaspoon onto griddles, close, and cook about 45 seconds until golden brown. The more you make the better you get at the exact amount of time to leave them on the iron. Peel off with a fork and let cool thoroughly on brown paper. Store in cardboard box lined with wax paper. Do not seal tight to avoid them getting soft.

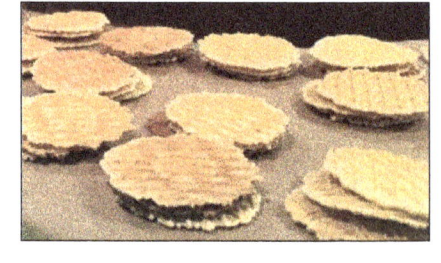

RUBY'S HEALTHY, EASY, AND COLORFUL PASTA SALAD
13 Net Carbs and 3 Fat
Serving size:1 cup

Ingredients
12 oz. box of whole wheat rotini
1 bag broccoli florets (trim and cut to bite sized)
1-pint grape tomatoes
1 red pepper (diced)
1 can pitted black olives (cut in half)
1 can chick peas (rinse and drain)
1 bag sun dried tomatoes (not in oil) chopped
1/2 16 oz. bottle of lite balsamic dressing (or to taste)

Directions
Cook pasta, drain, and toss in a small amount of Olive Oil to keep from sticking. While pasta cooks, combine all other ingredients in large bowl (lid preferred). Add entire bottle of dressing. Salt and pepper to taste. Add pasta once cooled and toss. Refrigerate overnight. Toss before serving.

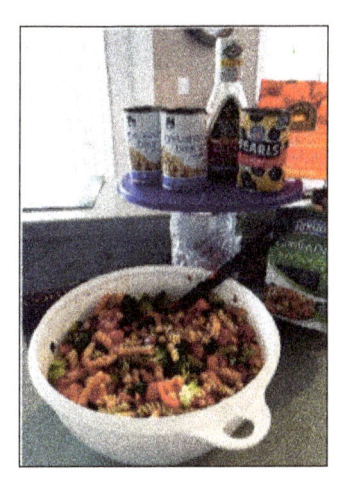

I have also added other fresh veggies if they're in my fridge, including carrots, celery, and fresh basil! Serves a lot! Recipe doubles very easy if you have a HUGE bowl.

Recipes that speak for themselves!
Losers Eat Good!

Influences on weight and body shape include biological, psychological, and cultural. Add to that disapproving messages and images of what a "healthy" person should look like. But we all come in a variety of shapes and sizes. That's why Losers works for so many people.

Chinese Carry Out & Delivery! Healthy choice chicken with mixed veggies over zero pasta! Track free!

LOSERS EAT GOOD!

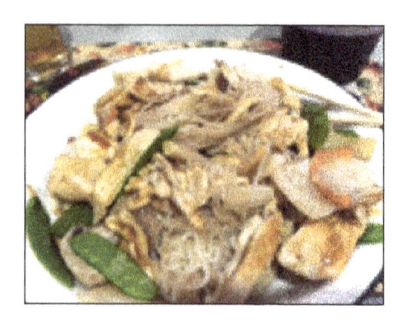

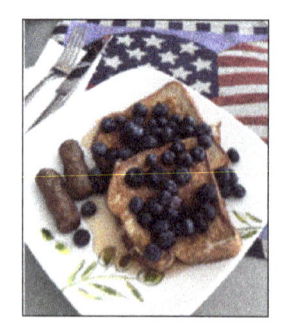

Breakfast at The Losers Café! Egg white French toast, turkey sausage, ½ cup fresh blueberries ¼ cup sugar free syrup. 27NC (including fruit) and 6Fat. Simply delicious.

WE EAT GOOD!

Polenta!! Four of these pieces have 15NC and 0Fat. We fry them with cooking spray and add some black pepper, and cayenne pepper!

YUMMY!

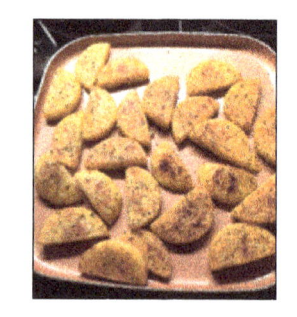

> You don't have to eat less, you just have to eat right.

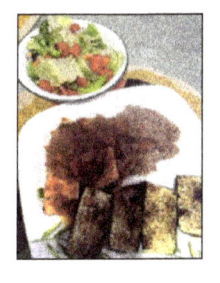

Salmon filets poached in salsa, grilled zucchini, one cup cooked bulgur wheat, and salad. 32NCs (30 is the bulgur wheat) & 2F.
WE EAT GOOD!

Pizza night on a single Joseph's Lavish bread. All lean protein, and veggies, ¼ cup of light mozzarella cheese. Track 7NC and 5Fat for the cheese.
MANGIAMO BENE!

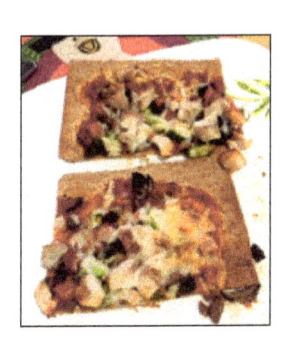

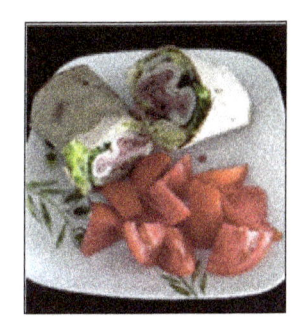

Lunch!! Deli turkey breast and roast beef on a Wellness wrap. Asiago Laughing Cow cheese as a bread spread. 6NC and 3Fats.
WE EAT GOOD!

Dinner at The Losers Café! Grilled Pork Chop (extra lean), grilled asparagus, sautéed Portobello mushrooms, and tomato-cucumber salad. Only had to track the Olive Oil on the salad: 5Fat.
WE EAT GOOD!

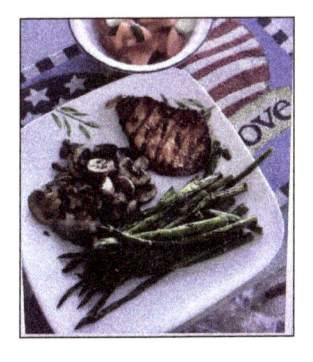

Track free! BBQ chicken and roasted asparagus and mushrooms cooked in the air fryer.
WE EAT GOOD!

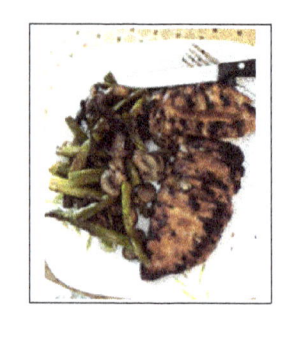

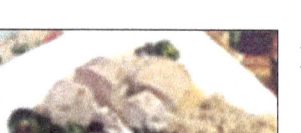

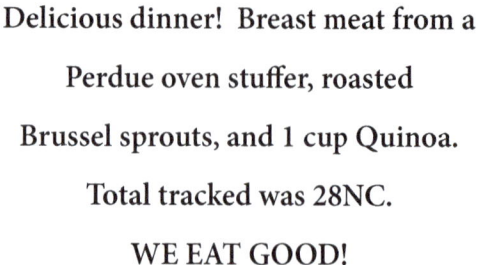

Delicious dinner! Breast meat from a Perdue oven stuffer, roasted Brussel sprouts, and 1 cup Quinoa. Total tracked was 28NC.
WE EAT GOOD!

Loser Surf & Turf! Grilled center cut pork chops, trimmed, steamed shrimp, and steamed cauliflower. 5NCs and 0Fat!
LOSERs EAT GOOD!

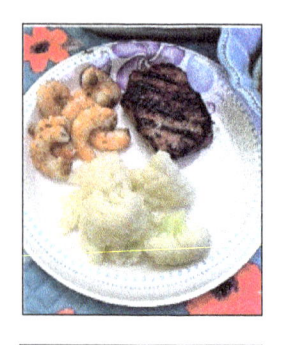

Chicken tenderloins sauteed with spinach, fresh mushrooms, and garden tomato. Nothing to track!! Use cooking spray to cook everything.
WE EAT GOOD!

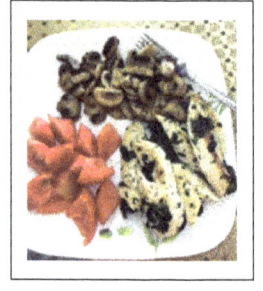

> Falling down is an accident,
> but staying down in a choice.

APPENDIX E

READ THE LABEL FIRST BEFORE YOU PUT IT IN YOUR MOUTH!

Compare labels to make sure you are getting the product with the lowest fat and NC.

Reminders:
- Net Carbs = Carbs minus Fiber
- 28grams = 1 ounce
- A 1-ounce serving of protein should be 2.5 grams of Fat or less.

Below is an example of a tracking day of various meals and snacks (the description of the meal is for information and is not part of a tracking chart). The example shows that for breakfast, only three of the five ingredients need to be tracked! Simple! Record your food and its grams of Net-Carbs and Fats.

> If you are serious, you will find a way.
> If you are not serious, you will find an excuse.

Food Item	Net Carb Grams	Fat Grams
Breakfast: a breakfast wrap with light string cheese, eggs, spinach, and some berries. Track only:		
Wellness Wrap	*5*	*1.5*
Cheese	*0*	*1.5*
1/2 cup blueberries	*9*	*0*
(mid morning snack) *Oikos Triple Zero Yogurt*	*9*	*0*
Lunch: Flatout wrap with Laughing Cow Light cheese used as bread spread. Lots of Turkey Breast and Roast Beef (reduced sodium from a deli) with lettuce and tomato. Small bag of Lay's Baked Chips. Track only:		
Wrap	*6*	*1.5*
Cheese	*1*	*1.5*
Chips	*18*	*3*
(afternoon snack) *small bag roasted edamame/soy beans*	*3*	*3*
Dinner: 2 grilled lean pork chops, roasted fresh asparagus, sauteed fresh mushrooms, 6-oz baked potato with 1 Tbs butter, salad with 2 Tbs Olive Garden Lite Dressing. Track only:		
Potato	*33*	*0*
Butter	*0*	*12*
Dressing	*2*	*2*
(evening snack) *Yasso Frozen Chocolate Chip Mint yogurt bar*	*14*	*1.5*
(evening snack) *16 animal crackers*	*23*	*2*
TOTAL	*123*	*29.5*

The following pages of this book are tracking pages to get you started. Duplicate as needed.

DAILY TRACKING FOR LOSERS

Food Item	Net Carb Grams	Fat Grams
TOTAL		

DAILY TRACKING FOR LOSERS

Food Item	Net Carb Grams	Fat Grams
TOTAL		

DAILY TRACKING FOR LOSERS

Food Item	Net Carb Grams	Fat Grams
TOTAL		

DAILY TRACKING FOR LOSERS

Food Item	Net Carb Grams	Fat Grams
TOTAL		

DAILY TRACKING FOR LOSERS

Food Item	Net Carb Grams	Fat Grams
TOTAL		

DAILY TRACKING FOR LOSERS

Food Item	Net Carb Grams	Fat Grams
TOTAL		

DAILY TRACKING FOR LOSERS

Food Item	Net Carb Grams	Fat Grams
TOTAL		

DAILY TRACKING FOR LOSERS

Food Item	Net Carb Grams	Fat Grams
TOTAL		

DAILY TRACKING FOR LOSERS

Food Item	Net Carb Grams	Fat Grams
TOTAL		

DAILY TRACKING FOR LOSERS

Food Item	Net Carb Grams	Fat Grams
TOTAL		

DAILY TRACKING FOR LOSERS

Food Item	Net Carb Grams	Fat Grams
TOTAL		

DAILY TRACKING FOR LOSERS

Food Item	Net Carb Grams	Fat Grams
TOTAL		

DAILY TRACKING FOR LOSERS

Food Item	Net Carb Grams	Fat Grams
TOTAL		

CPSIA information can be obtained
at www.ICGtesting.com
Printed in the USA
BVHW091045140119
537775BV00023B/3641/P

9 781628 062038